T0104861

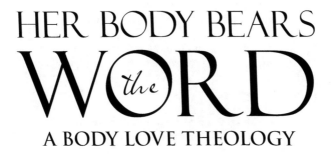

HER BODY BEARS
W*the*ORD
A BODY LOVE THEOLOGY

Jaimie D. Crumley

WESTBOW
P R E S S®
A DIVISION OF THOMAS NELSON
& ZONDERVAN

[Scripture quotations are] from the New Revised Standard Version
Bible, copyright © 1989 the Division of Christian Education of
the National Council of the Churches of Christ in the United
States of America. Used by permission. All rights reserved.

WestBow Press books may be ordered through
booksellers or by contacting:

WestBow Press
A Division of Thomas Nelson & Zondervan
1663 Liberty Drive
Bloomington, IN 47403
www.westbowpress.com
1 (866) 928-1240

ISBN: 978-1-5127-9343-7 (sc)
ISBN: 978-1-5127-9344-4 (e)

Library of Congress Control Number: 2017910693

Print information available on the last page.

WestBow Press rev. date: 07/20/2017

To my mother and my mothers.

CONTENTS

INTRODUCTION

HOW CAN THIS BE: GIVING OUR BODIES A THEOLOGY

Before we go any further, let's get one thing straight. The "perfect" female body is any female body that is prepared to be used by God. The premise of this book is that the female body is lovable and usable in the myriad forms in which it finds itself. As I write this book, I reflect on all the women I have known in my life. I have known women who were naturally curvaceous. I have known women who are naturally slender. I have known many women who were in-between. I have known women with athletic bodies. I have known women with significant physical challenges. I have known women who were in peak physical and mental condition and women who struggled with chronic illnesses and mental health issues. What most women I have known have in common is that their bodies change. Many women I know struggle to maintain a consistent weight or clear skin or peak mental health or perfect muscle definition or healthy skin, teeth, and nails. The only thing most of us maintain for most of our adult lives is our height, and even that is liable to change without notice! We often fight against these changes in our bodies. They are inconvenient, they are awkward, and sometimes they feel downright shameful. But lately, I have asked myself: why would God make us so dynamic if God could not use our dynamism to transform the world?

The question I bring with me to this work is: what kind of shape must my body be in for it to be usable for the work of God? It is at once an extremely personal question and a universal question. It is personal in that it is all about my body and what I need to do to get my body into God-shape. It is universal because we all have these bodies into which we were born. We all wrestle with these bodies. We all have things that we love about these bodies and things we despise about them. And as a Christian woman, I believe that each of our bodies were uniquely formed and created by God to serve God and the world. As a Christian woman, I also believe the sentence I just wrote is a complex statement because no two bodies are the same.

Some Christian writers have argued that God wants all of us to have the lowest body mass index possible, thus effectively shaming rounder bodies. Others have argued, in the words of the prophet Samuel, that people look at the outer appearance but God looks at the heart, thus effectively training Christians to neglect physical health (because it is only appearances, after all) in favor of developing a heart for God. I disagree with both of those stances. God is not in heaven judging our body mass indexes. God also would not have given us these physical bodies if they were about mere appearance. We are called to use these bodies to be good stewards of all of God's creation.

The time is now for us to release the body obsession so many of us have and to focus instead on love. Our outlooks change when we center our minds on love for God, love for self, and love for neighbors. I mean that deep, theological, earth-shattering, agape love that drives out fear. When we have that kind of love for our bodies, we don't fear weight gain, weight loss, roundness, flatness, thinness, flabbiness, or anything in between. Consider the adoption of a body love theology.

What is body love, and why does it matter? The truth is, I am a skinny girl writing about giving our bodies a theology. When I talk about body image or self-esteem, most people roll their eyes because I am naturally thin (which has come to be the beauty standard in much of the Western world), and I don't blame anyone for that reaction. However, since all of us have different bodies, we also all have a different body journey. We also must understand that our bodies are more than our physical appearance from the chin down. Our internal health and our mental health are to be tended to as well! My journey has been at once joyful, painful, confusing, and hopeful. Especially for women and girls, our bodies are constantly changing and are under constant scrutiny by everyone, from the people who love us the most to perfect strangers who pass us on the street.

Body-shaming is something women, from athletes to starlets to politicians to CEOs to teachers to pastors to housewives, have endured. Many women have shed light on their experiences in interviews, social media posts, books, and friend groups. Many other women have chosen to keep the trauma to themselves, often feeling too afraid to take a public stand. Regardless of our current shape and size, most of us have fantasized about life at a different shape and size. We have all endured insensitive comments about our weight. We have all grown frustrated with our bodies. We have all had moments that have caused us to confront head-on the reality that these bodies will one day expire.

Since I was in my late teens, even showing up to an exercise class invited commentary on my body shape, ranging from, "Why are you here?" to "I have been coming to this class for years; why don't I look like you?" As an adolescent, I loved eating, but I did not gain weight. During my elementary school years, my classmates pushed and shoved me and called me everything from ugly to anorexic. When I finally began to develop during my junior and senior years of high school and my metabolism began to slow down, I felt anxious. I didn't feel I fit in with the sporty, "skinny" girls because I had some curves, and the curves I had didn't exactly qualify me to call my frame curvy. As a black girl at a predominantly white school, I felt insecure about the body in which I suddenly existed, and at my predominantly black church on the weekends, I felt that somehow my body was not quite womanly enough.

By the time that I was a sophomore at my New England women's college, I was completely confused about this whole body confidence thing. I felt instinctively that the shape of my body didn't matter as much as my character and intelligence did. I also knew that while we technically should seek to get to know the people around us before deciding we already know them based on their physical appearance, first impressions include everything from clothing choices to hair to body types. Rarely do we have the opportunity to speak before being judged. At the time, that knowledge caused me to become physically, emotionally, and spiritually unhealthy. I began my journey to better health by relying on the all-sufficiency of God. As the years go by, I am learning to accept this body that God gave me and to choose to make it the healthiest version of itself that it can be. I am learning that this body of mine belongs to God. I am learning that God goes before me and girds me up on every side. So, I need to rely first on God and only then on what I offer physically, mentally, and emotionally.

I recognize that a conversation about something like body love or body positivity has a certain elitist ring to it. In many ways, it is a privilege held by women of means that we have disposable time to spend thinking about our bodies and how to mold them differently. For so many women all over the world, life is about survival. However, I would venture to say that we all are concerned about our bodies regardless of our means because we all inhabit bodies. I wish to write this text in such a way that we can take into serious consideration the bodies of those we render invisible every day, whoever they may be. Even if you are already a body positive woman, use this text as a tool to empower you to more deeply consider the bodies all over the world that, through our conscious and unconscious behaviors, are taught that they do not matter.

I try to cultivate a spirit of gratitude for having a body

that, although imperfect, functions at a high level without me even thinking about it. I celebrate having a body that can run and jump and dance but that also can rest and can sustain me for the journey ahead. So, when I say body positive, I mean body gratitude. I mean being grateful for what our bodies do and for what they do not do. I mean having gratitude for all our curves and all our edges. I mean being grateful for every break and tear and blemish, knowing that were created by a wonderful Creator.

I am a woman who grew up in the church. I treasure the words of Psalm 139 that teach me that I am "fearfully and wonderfully made." I don't ascribe to a cheap faith. Cheap faith says that we ought to accept being mistreated in this life because we are "children of the King." It is true that we Christians serve a marvelous Creator. It is also true that in Matthew 6, Jesus taught us to pray, saying, "Your kingdom come, Your will be done, on earth as it is in heaven." My reading of the Gospels teaches me that we must make earth like the kingdom of heaven. It teaches me that we don't passively accept the here and now, but rather that we strain to create a new here and now, a new heaven and a new earth. In this new heaven and new earth, I am judged by the times that I loved myself, my neighbors, and my community. I show love for myself by practicing self-care in everything, from the things I choose to put into my body to the things I choose to do with my body. I practice love for my neighbors by providing them with the tools to live their healthiest lives. I practice love for my community by keeping it healthy through my words, deeds, and actions. Our faith is insufficient if it doesn't do any work. My faith is insufficient if it does not love.

What is the power of the female physical form? In her hit 2011 song, "Who Run the World (Girls)," singer Beyoncé Knowles sings, "Boy, I know you love it. How we're smart enough to make these millions, strong enough to bear the children, then get back to business." Her provocative lyrics rang true to women from so many communities who are hardworking, smart, multidimensional, and multitalented. Furthermore, her lyrics assume male love for women's minds, work ethics, and bodies despite the history of violent male behavior toward bodies they perceive to be female. The boldness of her lyrics is a direct affront to the direct nature of male sexual aggression toward women when, if rebuffed, they say things like, "You know you love it." Her words turn such irresponsible and harmful words back onto the male listener, as he is bombarded by the power of a woman who knows who she is, what she wants, and what she has the capacity to achieve in the world. If that were not enough, the song proceeds to assert that female "persuasion can build a nation," which, even if not literally true, throughout history female bodies have birthed the nations and have sustained the lives of the nations. Her lyric is an affront to the notion that the nations have been built by male hands and male bodies and correctly identifies the female body as the source of any new human life that appears on the planet.

Knowles's music and brand have startled people from all walks of life from, the socially conservative who deem her to be irreverent, to devoted Christians who find her work to be counter to the tenets of Christian faith, to her peers in the music industry who are intimidated by her abilities as a singer and performer. Her presence has undeniably captivated the imaginations of an international audience. By no means do I intend to center her lyrics or image as representative of the Christian woman. I only center the lyrics because she inspires women, and many of the women and girls she impacts happen to be Christian. She has had a long-standing career in the entertainment industry that celebrates slimmer bodies, but she has a curvier frame and does nothing to obscure it. Even Knowles's choice to be a silent icon by no longer giving interviews on television or in magazines solidifies her power. She calls into question the reasons why women are silent. Perhaps the silent woman is not insecure or lacking in things to say. Instead, the silent woman is pondering, considering, holding onto her power. Perhaps that woman does what the Virgin Mary did when shepherds and angels came to glorify her newborn son. Perhaps a silent woman's power is held in her silence. Maybe that the female body in motion does not need so many words. The labor of her body is more than sufficient. Perhaps you do not need to spend so much time explaining your body to your world.

What would happen if we made the labor of the female body essential to our understanding of Christian theology? In the spring of 2014, when I was about halfway through my divinity school coursework, I had a dream. I am noting my educational journey because during the spring of 2014, my relationship to my education began to change. My parents first sent me to school as a two-year-old. I had been in an educational environment for the better part of the preceding twenty years of my life. I loved school. As a student, I knew what to do. I was not always a perfect student, but I knew the way the whole academic exercise was supposed to play out, and I played the part of the ideal student well, from the books that I carried, to my school supplies, to the way I dressed, to the way I sat. I knew the game. The problem is that I was getting older.

In the 2013–14 academic year, I had a part-time internship with a nonprofit parachurch organization in Hartford, Connecticut. My supervisor there was stretching me in new ways, and I was beginning to understand myself as more than a student. My experience with her was forcing me to rethink everything I had always believed to be true about myself. I was in my early twenties, and I was, for the first time, beginning to understand intellectually, socially, and spiritually what it meant that God had made me a woman called to Christian ministry. The deeper I dove into the pool of self-discovery, the more unsettled I became.

It was during this season of my life that I had a dream that forced me to confront my calling in a completely new way. I have always had vivid dreams, which are a constant source of frustration for me. I figure that if I lead a perfectly productive day, I should not be forced to have dreams so vivid that when I awake, I feel like I have not gotten any sleep at all. However, when I take a step back from my human desire to feel well-rested, I understand my dreams to be a subconscious way to revealing to me the things that ought to matter most to me. Dreams reveal what I cannot see in the hustle and bustle of day-to-day life. Dreams have the power to change the way we see ourselves and our world. I had such a dream that night in 2014.

In the dream, there were lots of synchronized swimmers, all young women, who were swimming in perfect coordination. Meanwhile, two women sat in chairs right next to the pool, watching the women as they dove and spun and turned and danced with perfect synchronicity. The women did not swim because one of them was extremely pregnant and the other was there to look after her; she could go into labor at any moment. The two women outside the pool chatted and sipped on lemonade as they watched the other women swim. They were at once fully engrossed in their interaction with one another and deeply intrigued by the beauty of the swimmers.

Suddenly, the pregnant woman's water broke, and it was if the synchronized swimmers had forgotten how to swim. They flew recklessly into the water, bashing their heads on the bottom of the pool and colliding with each other. It was a disaster! Meanwhile, an ambulance rushed to the scene to take the pregnant woman to the hospital. Paramedics jumped out of the ambulance to help her. The woman who was there to look after her kept her eyes focused on her charge. Neither the women getting into the ambulance nor the paramedics seemed to have any regard for the bloody mess unfolding all around them. The goal that day was to care for the woman who was now in labor, and no one would be distracted from that task. My dream ended there. I did not get to see the pregnant young woman's new child, nor did I get to see what became of the chaos in the pool.

My dream that night astounded me. The sight of these young, talented synchronized swimmers completely losing control of their abilities to do the thing they had done so beautifully just a moment before terrified me. Likewise, the sight of this woman, heavy with child, suddenly going into labor next to the pool confused me. The fact that neither the pregnant woman's caregiver nor the paramedics who rushed to the scene to care for her paid any heed to the gruesome scene that was rapidly unfolding in the pool disrupted my spirit. Yes, this bringing this new life into the world was important, but how could everyone ignore all the lives being destroyed in the pool? I believed I had a dream about a great tragedy, a tragedy in which perfect women fell out of sync with one another and became imperfect all because of the change happening with their sister's body.

I started talking to those closest to me about the dream. I didn't know what to make of it, so I needed someone else to interpret it for me. Many of my interpreters provided beautiful understandings of who the women could be. They asked me if perhaps I was one of the women in the pool. Others were sure that I was the woman who was disrupting the order by giving birth to a new thing. One wondered whether I was the woman charged to care for the pregnant woman and that perhaps the dream was revealing that I needed to stay focused on the one thing God had given me to care for and trust that the women in the pool could regain their synchronicity. I was disturbed by that last interpretation. I felt that the interpretation indicated that I was selfish or myopic. I also felt a bit useless because the women in the pool used their bodies as things of beauty, and the woman giving birth was producing a new life, but the body of the woman that might represent me did nothing but sit around and wait. I wondered why these two women were even at the pool that day. Sure, they might have been associated with the swimmers, but considering the situation, couldn't they have sat together somewhere else? The more answers I received, the more questions emerged.

My natural tendency is to operate in a task-oriented manner. I consider a task that needs completion and I think through the necessary steps to complete the task. So, when I initially had this dream, the reason I was so concerned was because the women in the pool were not properly completing their task. I wondered why the natural bodily actions of one woman outside of their situation prevented their progress. I have come to understand through sitting more with the dream and from being influenced by the ministry of people who taught me that my body was an asset that my theology must operate as though women's bodies mattered. More specifically, the dream shifted my imagination when it comes to the study of God. Suddenly I realized that theology is not theology if it is unconcerned with the needs of the human body. The dream indicated that the flourishing of the female body is more important than the completion of practical tasks. Perhaps I needed to understand even that my body matters because God made it. Since that dream, my work has shifted. I challenge both myself and my readers or listeners to understand that women's minds, bodies, and spirits are central to the completion of the work God is doing in our world.

We know that the female body is of supreme importance

to God because scripture indicates as much. Many of the named female characters in scripture are defined by their reproductive abilities. Many of the writers of the Bible erred in their comprehension of women because they viewed women as merely reproduction machines. As a contemporary Christian woman, I shudder at the idea. We must read deeper than the words on the page; we have to read using the eyes of the Holy Spirit. Rereading those same stories of barrenness turned to fruitfulness through a renewed hermeneutical lens allows us to see that God loves women because God gave women the most essential job of creation—that is, with great pain to become cocreators with God. That said, God values women's bodies even when they do not reproduce. Plenty of women in scripture are named without mention of any children they might have birthed. Deborah in Judges was a woman of great import to Israel, and we never read of any husband or children. Mary and Martha are known by their friendship with Jesus and their siblinghood with Lazarus and one another. Phoebe is known for her great assistance within the church. Countless other women in scripture and throughout human history have used their bodies to "bear the Word," even without ever physically bearing a child. Even when our bodies are not engaged in this task of cocreation, they maintain beauty, elegance, and mystery that is beyond words. It is for that reason that throughout the history of the world, women's bodies have been feared, misunderstood, and abused instead of celebrated. Even in female-only spaces, these attitudes are reinforced, perhaps even more strongly, because of our fundamental misunderstandings of our own bodies.

By no means am I an expert on health or the human body. However, as I think back about that dream I had years ago, I am coming to understand that I have something to say about the theology of body love. Certainly, there is no Christian theology that can call itself Christian and be unconcerned with the human body. For, in the beginning, God formed the human frame from the dust of the earth and breathed life into it. God is intimately acquainted with the human body, and God contains us within these human bodies until the day our spirits take their eternal rest.

In this book, I focus specifically on the labor and pain of being cocreators with God. While this book is a body love theology that has been written specifically bearing in mind those who are anatomically female, the concepts in the book are for all bodies. As I pointed out in the preceding paragraph, God took great care in creating the human form. This book merely focuses on those born in female bodies because of the shame placed upon women both within and outside of the Christian tradition when our bodies in some way fail to conform to a social norm. I hope readers will derive a few lessons from this book. First, listen to your body because it has a story to tell. Second, celebrate your body because as the Psalmist wrote, it is fearfully and wonderfully made. Finally, make your body work for you; it a beautiful vessel that can better society.

By the end of this book, I hope you marvel at the possibilities of your body, not because it is a perfect body but because it is a functional body that can be used as a tool for change in the world. Our bodies endure so many thoughtless misdeeds during their sojourn on earth, so I wonder in this text how we can come to better love and care for these bodies. We can all be filled with wonder when it comes to these bodies, and our spiritual imaginations must expand so that we recognize what is going on when angels appear in our lives, calling on us to live out our callings in new ways. May we say in those moments, as Mary did, "How can this be?" And then, may we be prepared to take on the challenges that are ahead, knowing that God has prepared us for such a time as this. You, your beautiful body, and your curious soul are about to change the world because, with God, nothing will be impossible.

Prayer: Lord, I am trusting You as I embark on this new journey toward a theology of body love. Through this journey, I pray that You will open me to the possibilities of my body. Teach me to embrace every curve and every edge. Teach me to reach toward health. Teach me to use my body as a creative tool. Provide me with the tools to use my body as an instrument for You and to help others to do likewise. God, this broken vessel belongs to You. Thank You for creating me. Amen.

CHAPTER 1

EVE BORE SETH TO REPLACE ABEL (GENESIS 4:25)

*H*ave you ever noticed how terrifying Eve's story is? Her life went from literal perfection to sheer terror in a matter of nineteen verses of scripture! Here's what I see: I see a woman created to be with a man as his partner. Life was perfect for them at first. There was plenty to eat and to drink. Their only job was to take care of a completely unblemished world. They sang with birds, swam with fish, and spoke with serpents. In addition, they did not have to worry at all about fashion. God had created this first man and woman in bodies that they deemed were functional enough for survival. They roamed the earth unashamedly naked. We are given no indication about whether their bodies were flat or round or tall or short. All we know is that they were naked bodies, ready to take on their lives.

One day, Eve made the mistake of talking to the wrong serpent. And why would she not talk to every serpent who passed by and struck up a conversation? She had no reason to be suspicious of serpents, or any other living thing for that matter, because she did not know anything about sin. The serpent had a bright new idea for Eve, which was that Eve could eat from the only tree from which God had explicitly forbidden them to consume. The tree was rather descriptively called the tree of the knowledge of good and evil. Eve considered eating from the tree but quickly retorted that she could not. God had told Adam and Eve that if they ate from that tree, they would die. I wonder what Eve thought it meant to die. Her life was perfect, so it is no wonder the possibility of death had kept her curiosity at bay. Who would want to leave paradise? Despite Eve's protest, the serpent persisted and piqued Eve's interest. For the first time, she realized disobeying God was an option. The serpent told her that the reason why God wanted to keep her away from the tree was that eating from the tree would allow her to become like God, knowing all good and all evil.

Now here is where we usually start judging Eve. How many times have you heard a preacher or Sunday school teacher take a judgmental, lecturing tone when Eve becomes interested in the possibilities of sin? Normally, the teacher or preacher places his or her hand on his or her hip and says something like, "Now Eve had her pick of every tree in the garden, but she just had to eat that fruit. She just had to be disobedient." And those preachers and teachers have a point. Sin was Eve's choice. Why would she choose sin when living without sin was so perfect? There was nothing she lacked. She had full access to everything a good father gives his children. Eve chose disobedience at that moment, and that is objectional.

However, when we do serious self-examination, we understand that this story of Eve is the human story. Eve's story directly mirrors the way that all of us first discover sin. Our desire to sin is sparked by genuine curiosity. We wonder what would happen if we forged our own paths. Our choice is sparked by a genuine thirst for knowledge. It is sparked by our sudden realization of our own mortality, the realization that these bodies are not forever. In that moment of realization, we decide that we must immediately know everything, see everything, and understand everything before it is too late. Our ambition overtakes us. So, overwhelmed by her irresistible curiosity, Eve opened her mouth and consumed that which God had told her should never enter her body, and her life was forever changed.

Can you relate? Have you ever made a choice that forever altered the course of your life because you were too ambitious to do otherwise? Sometimes these choices of ours are completely divinely appointed, but other times, these choices reflect our tendency to do what is right in our own eyes. Eve's decision points to a certain mystery of women. Intellectually, Eve knew what God had told her to do, and she was committed to obedience. The problem then is that she was spirited, she was curious, and she was creative. In that moment of spirited, creative curiosity, she forever reshaped the human story. For better or for worse, we are who we are because of the eating habits of one spirited, creative, and curious woman. A woman's hunger has birthed us.

The so-called fall from grace story teaches us that that one spirited, creative, curious, hungry woman transformed the social and physical demands of womanhood through her disobedience. She teaches us something about the relationship between food and our bodies. What we eat literally and philosophically influences the people we are. Her actions support the idea that you are what you eat. Her action is a reminder that we honor and dishonor God even by the way we eat.

God never deprived Adam and Eve, but God did set limits on their eating habits. As Christians, we believe that no food is unclean but the belief that no food is unclean is not then an instruction that we must eat everything. How would our lives be different if we sought to honor God, even in our eating habits, knowing that what we eat influences our relationship with God? The answer to that question is completely different for each one of us. I am not advocating any one diet as being holier than any other; rather, I am wondering what dietary plan best reflects your relationship with your Creator.

When Eve ate from the tree of the knowledge of good and evil, everything changed for her and Adam. For one thing, the man and the woman realized for the first time that they were unclothed, and they stitched together fig leaves to cover themselves. Where their nakedness had once represented their innocent vulnerability with one another, it now represented the possibility of carnal sin. The opening of their eyes to all sin is a reminder that the choices we make, whether good or bad, influence every other aspect of our lives. Once our eyes are open to a new way of life, we see all of it: the good and the bad.

In Genesis 3:16, we learn that Eve's punishment for consuming fruit from the tree of the knowledge of good and evil was that God would "greatly increase [her] pangs in childbearing; in pain [she] shall bring forth children, yet [her] desire shall be for [her] husband, and he shall rule over [her]." That statement is an effective discouragement from getting married and having children! Before this point, I wonder if Eve had even been aware of the reproductive possibilities of her body. Because of her sin, she was also going to become well acquainted with the pain of bringing new life into the world. With that, Adam and Eve were driven out of the garden because they now knew the difference between good and evil. They had sacrificed paradise for a piece of fruit.

Since Adam and Eve's expulsion from Eden, bearing children has become part of the fabric of human life. It is understood to be something that women's bodies simply do. In making bearing children such a normal, and even expected, part of the human experience, we have failed to appreciate fully the wonder of the work God does in women's bodies to create new life. God has chosen women to become cocreators with God through the pain of childbirth. It is an astounding miracle that the female body is built to facilitate the recreation of humanity in the world. It is astounding that female bodies sustain unborn children. Female bodies grow and shift to accommodate new life, and then they bear the new life into the world through pain and groaning. God could bring new life into the world in a million different ways, but the female reproductive system is the way God chose.

So how did it feel to be the first woman to feel that shift in her body? To this day, we hear phrases like "[Woman's name] is the first woman to ever do/win/

achieve [accomplishment]." Many of us know what it feels like to be or to know the first woman ever to accomplish a given thing. At first blush, it seems like an honor to be the first woman to have made a significant or historical achievement. It feels like the first woman is opening the door for many more women to flood in behind her. But it also feels like a slap in the face, doesn't it? Why is it that in the twenty-first century there are still doors that women are walking through for the first time? Why do so many doors remain closed to women? Why is it that women still must prove our strength, our intellect, our courage, and our potential? There are many ways to answer that question, and my goal is not to get us bogged down in attempting to answer it. My goal is only to say that many women living today have been the first, will be the first, or know the first. We stand where Eve stood, feeling a new thing stir within us for the first time. We know the discomfort that newness causes in everyone around us. We know the anxiety new beginnings arouse in us.

Eve was, or at least she represents, the world's first human mother. What did it feel like to be the first woman who started looking strange to everyone around her because she was growing in new and unexpected ways? Eve must have even looked strange to herself. God had hinted at this childbearing thing before her expulsion from Eden, but she could not have known that women bear children into the world by carrying them in their wombs for nine months. God had warned Adam and Eve about this "pain in childbirth" thing, but how did they know how pregnancy was going to look? Who did Eve turn to when she needed to determine how to care for herself in this time of immense change? There were no older women, no sisters, and no midwives. What are we without mentors and role models? I wonder what it felt like when she experienced those first little kicks in her womb. And I wonder what it felt like to endure that pain of childbirth not really understanding what it meant. What does it feel like to you when you feel or see a change in your body that no one else can see or explain? I get stomachaches often. Sometimes they are easily explainable, and at other times, they seem to have been brought on by nothing. In those moments, I have been taught by spiritual leaders I know to check in with my body to determine how I can attend to it. I have found that those stomach pains usually relate to some need around me or some longing of my soul. But Eve did not have anyone to teach her. She had to rely on the signs provided to her by her Creator.

The scripture gives us no indication of what Eve might have endured socially, physically, emotionally, or spiritually during her pregnancy. All we know for sure is that she did endure, and we know that because she gave birth to three sons. I would venture to say that in those days, Eve had such a connected relationship with God that she could trust God to take care of her body. So, if it was changing rapidly and unexpectedly, perhaps she chose not to be afraid because she knew that God created her mystery of a body. Her silence in the face of radical physical change makes me wonder what our lives would look like if we surrendered our bodies fully to God. What would it look like if women and men allowed our bodies to go through changes unselfconsciously, knowing that if our bodies were changing, it indicated that perhaps God was doing a new thing with and through us, that maybe we could come to understand the change in its perfect time?

Then there was the pain. Although scripture does not explicitly state it, I imagine that in the garden of Eden, no one felt any pain. But now, they were in the real world. Adam toiled and sweat; he knew what pain was. Eve managed the burdens of work around the house; she knew what pain was. But this kind of pain was something Eve was not fully prepared to encounter. This pain was the pain that God warned Eve about. This was a punishing pain. Eve bore the full, crushing weight of what it meant to be a Creator. Her experience teaches us about the deep pain God endures to produce the entirety of creation. Great beauty is born through anguish. Eve's childbearing pain introduced new life into the world. This was the kind of pain that introduced life that would sometimes fall short of the glory of God. This was the kind of pain that produced children who would, at one time or another, break their Creator's heart. In that moment of childbirth, Eve physically endured the pain that her Creator must have felt, gazing upon her and Adam that day in the garden, covered in fig leaves.

Eve's body bore immense pain to bring two imperfect boys into the world. And for me, that's the rub. What happens when we endure the physical pain, and it seems like our only prize, for that endurance is a different kind of pain? What then? We know the story. Eve gave birth to two sons. First, Cain, a gardener, and second, Abel, a shepherd. Cain had an anger problem. God accepted his brother's offering but had no regard for his offering. People always ask, "Well, why didn't God accept Cain's offering?" but that is not the point. The objective is to show us that Adam and Eve passed on sin to the next generation. If we had perhaps hoped that humanity's sin problem would end with Adam and Eve, allowing future generations to return to paradise, we had hoped in vain. In Genesis 4:7 God encouraged Cain to master his strong temptation to sin. It is the first time in the Bible that we learn that we can consider sin but choose otherwise. We are the masters of our sinful natures. But Cain does not master his sinful nature, and he kills his brother in the field. God put a mark on Cain so no one would hurt him and sent him away into the land of Nod, east of Eden.

Now, Eve had endured the physical pain of bringing both of her sons into the world. She raised them. She ran and played with them in their childhood, made sure they never went hungry, fed them, clothed them, gave them shelter, and for what? One of them was dead, and the other was driven out of town. Her body bore them, nurtured them, and sustained them, and just like that, they were gone. And the only thing we hear about her after she gave birth to Cain and Abel comes in Genesis 4:25, when she gave birth to another son and named him Seth, because he was replacing Abel. The verse has always clung to me eerily. Eve had one murdered son, one banished son, and the only thing we hear about her in response is that she decided to have a replacement son.

I don't get it! Her boys had messed up. They had let her down. They had hurt her deeply. And they weren't coming back. And her response was to try again. As my mother reminded me recently, failing and choosing to try again anyway is the way we survive (and thrive) in life. We are dealt blows over the course of our lives that seem unfair, that threaten to break us, that devastate us. The measure of our character is whether we get up, dust ourselves off, regroup, trust God, and continue to live. And in the face of the greatest tragedy a mother could be forced to endure, the loss of both of her children, Eve chose to get up, to dust herself off, to regroup, to reconnect with the life partner God had given her, to trust God, and to choose life. And for Eve, choosing life looked like bearing another child, considering him a gift from God, and loving him with all her heart.

Eve bore a replacement son named Seth. Today's psychological theories would tell us that it is something a parent should never do. I would like to think that Eve took time for herself, for her own health, to cultivate her relationship with her partner, and then made this decision. scripture does not tell us what Eve did to care for herself in the interim between the loss of Cain and Abel and the birth of Seth. What we do know, however, is that Eve loved Seth. What we also know is that as the world's first mother, the experience with Cain and Abel probably made Eve a better mother to her son Seth. She could be a better teacher for him about sin, grace, and hope than she ever was to Cain and Abel. Failure has a way of molding us for the better.

In time, Seth married and had his own child. Humankind came to be, and these humans began to know God. Future generations came to understand that despite their sin, God's grace toward them abounded.

Eve's story disturbs the deepest parts of my soul, I think because it rings so true. Our bodies succeed, and they fail. Our labors can bring us such delight, and they can bring us such pain. If Eve's story teaches us anything, it is to continue to push our bodies, believing in their abilities to bring us the kind of joy that outweighs the tragedies. Eve did not have Seth as a replacement for Abel. No, she believed that God gave her Seth. What gifts will God give you if you release the traumas of your past to bring new things into the world? Can your deepest shame create an opening for your greatest blessing?

Prayer: Dear Lord, I confess that I am a sinner. Thank You for your grace that abounds toward me. I thank You that despite my sin, You call me Your own. Lord, even as I explore the fullness of my spirited, creative, and curious nature, remind me to place You at the center of any choice I make. And Lord, as You do new things in me for which I have no roadmap, teach me to be still, and to place my trust in You. Amen.

CHAPTER 2

REBEKAH BORE CONFLICTED NATIONS: GENESIS 25:21–28

*T*his book is not about God miraculously opening the wombs of barren women. I do not have any children, and only time will tell whether I will or not. What I do know, however, is that many women throughout world history have suffered because of infertility and from not being able to carry their children to term. Like the women whose stories are lifted in scripture, many of these women pray for God's help. For some, they find a remedy, and for others, it seems there is no remedy. Barrenness or never having had children is not a curse; it does not make one less of a woman, nor does it point to a physical flaw. Struggling with fertility is the reality for lots of women, and according to many statistics on the topic, many women in my generation will never have a child in their lives. Childbearing is not what makes a woman a woman. But for generations of women, society has led them to believe that childbearing defines womanhood. So, when I write about pregnancies in this book, even of women who were once barren, I don't want to make their barrenness the central topic.

Unfortunately, scripture refuses to allow me to conveniently side step the reality that so many of the women whose pregnancies scripture focuses on happened to have issues with conceiving and that God opened their wombs. One response to such a view of women's wombs is that pregnancy in scripture is always about more than just pregnancy or being accepted by men and society. For the women in the Bible, childbearing gave an entry in the mystical club of mothers. But childbearing was about more than just social standing with other women. It was an entry into some sort of political relevance. The barren women we meet in scripture proceed to give birth to prophets, patriarchs, and new nations. These women become the mothers of great promise. By the power of the Holy Spirit, human experience has progressed in much of the developed world when it comes to women (although I would say that more evolution is certainly needed). Today, feminist theory, womanist thought, and historical precedent teach us that a woman's body can be the source of prophecy, social leadership, and political change. These are products that she can produce out of her abilities, intellect, and skill, not just through having children.

In this chapter, I want to focus on Rebekah's pregnancy. Like Eve, Rebekah was a woman whose story was told in the Hebrew Bible. Unlike Eve, she would have known plenty of women who became mothers before she did. Rebekah was the wife of Isaac, and Isaac was the son of Abraham and Sarah, the great patriarch and matriarch of the children of Israel. You might remember that God had promised Abraham and Sarah a son and that they had given up all hope because in Sarah's old age, they still did not have a child. But God had promised Abraham and Sarah a son, and they had one and called him Isaac. No doubt Isaac had his challenges during his childhood. For one thing, his father, Abraham, had laid him on an altar in the wilderness like a ram to sacrifice him to God, but God spared him from a gruesome and untimely death at the last minute. For another thing, it could not have been easy to be the son of parents who were advanced in age and life experience. I imagine it might also have been a challenge to bear the weight of all their hopes on his shoulders. As an only child, I understand that pressure in part, but I imagine it must have been almost unbearable for Isaac. He was a child of divine promise. We do not get insight into Isaac's inner struggles because unlike his father Abraham and his son Jacob he took more of a passive role in the formation of the new nation of God's chosen people.

Silent Isaac was married to a woman who was anything but silent. Much like Eve, she was spirited, creative, and curious to a fault. She had a personal relationship with God, but for some reason, she did not seem to have received the good news that God could carry out a divine plan without her intervention. In Genesis 24, we learn about the beginnings of their relationship. Isaac began his life with Rebekah after his mother, Sarah, had died, and his father, Abraham, was advanced in years. Since Isaac was the only child of Abraham and Sarah, Abraham felt it was urgent to find him a partner. He refused to allow his son to return to his homeland but did not want him to have a Canaanite wife. Abraham had a servant swear an oath to find Isaac a wife from his homeland and to attempt to bring her back into the land that God had promised Abraham and his descendants. So, the servant went out, taking with him all sorts of gifts from Abraham, to find the woman who would leave her family and homeland behind to settle with Isaac in Canaan. The servant brought the camels to kneel by a well outside of the city of Nahor, which was the region near the upper Euphrates River. As he and the camels rested near the well, a beautiful young woman named Rebekah approached and offered water, not only to the servant but the camels as well. Culturally, this was viewed as an act of hospitality, and the servant knew at that moment that Rebekah was the woman he sought. As a further sign of not only Rebekah's hospitality but also of the hospitality of her family, they provided overnight lodgings for the servant and his camels.

After hearing the servant's story, they agreed to allow Rebekah to return to Canaan to be Isaac's wife. One interesting part of Rebekah's story is the amount of agency her family gave her in the situation. No doubt, the agreement that she should marry a man she had never met is paternalistic. But this family ultimately shows their respect for the young, newly betrothed woman. When the servant and the camels awakened after their overnight stay with Rebekah's family, the servant was ready to leave and take Rebekah with him. Many stories in scripture show families essentially discarding unmarried women and girls to the first available suitor. Not so with Rebekah's family. They requested an additional ten days with her. When the servant insisted that he could not wait, they called her and asked her whether she would go with the servant, and after she had agreed, they allowed her to go. Even in a powerless situation, this family found a way to empower their girl, and we later see her exercise that empowered spirit her family had cultivated in her while she was raising her sons. Rebekah went to Canaan and became Isaac's partner and wife, a comfort to him after the loss of his mother.

This empowered woman's story is the driving force of this story. She was at once the submissive wife and the scheming young woman, eager to aid the work God in the work God was doing in her family even though God never asked for her help. Her barrenness is part of the plot line, but only barely. Rebekah could have been like many women throughout the history of time for whom becoming pregnant is not an easy task. Perhaps she was not barren. Rather, maybe her body was not yet ready to produce new life and did so in its own time. In Genesis 25:21, we learn that Isaac prayed for Rebekah because she was barren and that the Lord answered Isaac's prayer and Rebekah conceived. Perhaps all many women need to be empowered to be cocreators with God is partners who are committed to prayer.

When Rebekah finally conceived, she was carrying twins, and the babies waged a fierce war inside her womb. Even as I write, I feel a battle raging inside of me because I am human. We humans are not monolithic creatures. Just think about all we have going on with our identities. We have a gender, race or ethnicity, age, ability level, sexual orientation, and social class. Those social identifiers do not even begin to account for our theologies, families, professions, or personal interests. We all have a lot going on! Social science scholars call the phenomenon of having a variety of social identities that converge to create one person "intersectionality." In their 2016 book, *Intersectionality*, Patricia Hill Collins and Sirma Bilge define intersectionality as "a way of understanding and analyzing the complexity of the world, in people, and in human experiences."[1] It is true, the world we live in has constructed these social structures, and we certainly have the option not to accept any of them, but we at least must acknowledge their presence. They affect everything, from the way we perceive the world around us and the way the world perceives us in return. Personally, my social identity even impacts the way I approach the study of scripture. The intersectionality of my existence sometimes causes me to physically or emotionally react to things that are happening in the world, sometimes without even being able to verbally render meaning to my reaction.

I introduce the concept of intersectionality because I think Rebekah might have been the first woman we encounter in scripture to wrestle with the reality of intersectionality although she did not have the words to articulate it. Her body felt it acutely. Her body bore a fiercely intersectional identity. When Rebekah gave birth, she bore two sons, twins. What is it to give birth to twin children who at every level are at odds with one another? Her first son was red and hairy, so they named him Esau. The name signals Esau's ancestry of Edom, and the Hebrew word *se'ar* (hairy) echoes the word Seir, which was a region of Edom. Her second son emerged

---

[1] Patricia Hill Collins and Sirma Birge. (2016) *Intersectionality,* Malden, MA: Poly Press. 1.

gripping his brother's heel, so they called him Jacob or *ya'aqov* in Hebrew, which is motivated by the word *'aqev*, the Hebrew word for heel.[2]

Much has been made of Rebekah's aid to her trickster son Jacob when she believed that he was the rightful inheritor of Isaac's blessing. However, little is made of the experience within Rebekah's body as she carried a pair of feuding twins in her womb. Unlike Eve's pregnancy, Rebekah's pregnancy sounds traumatic. We learn that she indeed felt the pains of the changes happening within her body, and she even wonders in verse 22 why she remained alive through all the pain. Has your body ever gone through physical changes that caused you so much pain or discomfort that you wondered why you were even alive? Some of my friends who suffer from chronic reproductive illnesses like endometriosis have told me about the debilitating pain and the trauma that happens in their bodies because of their ailment.

Many of us are familiar with the sort of physical pain that feels like it might devour us from the inside out. Because of the way that God created the female body, many women are more acutely familiar with the sort of pain that Rebekah might have felt as she was preparing to bring her sons Esau and Jacob into the world. But it is important for us to remember that this pain was unique to Rebekah. The reality is that as much as we empathize with one another's aches and pains and traumatic experiences,

---

[2] Attridge, Harold W, Wayne A. Meeks (Eds.) (2006) *The HarperCollins study Bible: New Revised Standard Version, with the Apocraphal/Deuterocanonical Books* San Francisco, Calif.: HarperSanFrancisco, 40.

we do not live in each other's bodies. Our experiences of pain and trauma are not monolithic. Your pains are your pains, the changes in your body are the changes in your body. While another person might be able to come alongside you and relate to you and share the journey with you, we are all on our own paths to wholeness. So, as Rebekah cried out to God, "Why do I live?" she was tending to her aches and pains through her spiritual connection with God. The way she expresses her anguish in response to the pain within her body is not for us to judge or correct; it is simply for us to accept. This was Rebekah's bone to pick with God, and by the grace of God, she was provided with the assurance she needed that her pain had a purpose.

We are then introduced to a motif that becomes a theme in the Hebrew Bible, the youngest son who rules over his older brothers. The twin boys Rebekah carried in her womb struggled even there because the younger son was a threat to everything society said the older son should be. He was the leader. He was the ruler. And the elder brother would serve him. Perhaps the younger brother sought to switch places with his older brother so they would not even have to entertain the problem. But to no avail. Even in the womb, Esau was physically stronger, but Jacob was wilier. Rebekah literally gave birth to conflicting personalities, Esau, a skillful hunter who loved the fields, and Jacob, a quieter, cultured man who lived in tents. And Isaac loved Esau because he was fond of meat, and Rebekah loved her younger son, Jacob. And so, through one woman's body, the story of Israel was born.

Prayer: Dear Lord, I give You every part of who I am so I can be used for You. Help me to endure the pain of bringing new things into the world. Help me to love more fully the gifts that You have given me. Lord, give me the tools to diminish social barriers between people that we all might live in peace. Amen.

CHAPTER 3

ELIZABETH BORE GREAT MERCY: LUKE 1:24–25, 57–58

*I*n chapter 6 we will talk more about Mary, the mother of Jesus. Mary was a young virgin who learned that she was going to be the God-bearer. She, better than anyone else, teaches us that our bodies are made in service to God, and that God can (and will) use any body God deems fit. This chapter is not about Mary. No, this chapter is about an older woman, Mary's cousin, Elizabeth, who was Mary's spiritual midwife. Elizabeth was in a loving marriage to a priest named Zechariah. Elizabeth was held in high esteem around town. Luke 1:5 says that she was a descendant of Aaron. Do you remember Aaron? We meet Aaron in the book of Exodus. He was the cousin of Moses, and he served as the priest to the children of Israel during their long journey to the Promised Land. He was a key player in the spiritual formation of Israel.

Zechariah and Elizabeth were respected for more than their sacred lineage. Luke 1:6 says, "Both of them were righteous before God, living blamelessly according to all the commandments and regulations of the Lord." Zechariah and Elizabeth were not the type of folks who rested on their laurels. They spent their time trying to live in ways that were worthy of the awesome call that God had placed on both of their lives. I imagine that they would have been known for caring for their neighbors, loving children who were not their own, volunteering for the jobs no one else wanted to do, visiting prisoners, and caring for the sick. They were pillars of their community.

But this holy couple had a rather embarrassing problem that had plagued them throughout their marriage. Their problem was embarrassing because they could not hide it. There is really something particularly painful about public shame. It is one thing to have problems we can keep to ourselves, the illnesses we can live with quietly, the unsuccessful job interviews no one knows we went to, the addiction we are so sure we are hiding from the rest of the world. But this problem was obvious, and it became more embarrassing with each passing year. Zechariah and Elizabeth could do as many wonderful things around town as they wanted to, but everyone whispered behind their backs anyway.

Their great embarrassment was that Elizabeth was barren, and they were getting on in years. Like Rebekah, the subject of the preceding chapter, Elizabeth was ashamed. The great irony of the shame of women who struggle with fertility is that especially in ancient times (and often now as well) women bear the brunt of that shame. Never in scripture do we see any consideration given to the idea that perhaps a woman's fertility has little or nothing to do with a failure of her reproductive system.

However, let's just follow the tone of the story line which indicates that if a woman is barren, it is due to a failing of her body.

Elizabeth was a woman who clearly transformed her community, who spoke words of healing to those who needed them most, and who cared for the sick and the needy. That woman's body was doing work that was more than sufficient, and yet, society was teaching her to be ashamed because her body had not done the one thing everyone thought a woman's body ought to do. A friend who has gotten into yoga over the past few years tells me that one of the most important lessons she has learned from her practice is to consider the successes and the limitations of her body nonjudgmentally. She tells me that approaching her body with this mind-set has allowed her to grow into greater body acceptance and to make whatever adjustments she needs to make to have a healthier body from a place of love rather than from a place of condemnation. One of the most important things we can do for our bodies is to be honest about their strengths and their limitations without judgement or shame. We are healthier when we approach our bodies from places of love and acceptance. There is grace and beauty even in the things that the world says should bring us shame. Elizabeth found it impossible to approach her infertility nonjudgmentally.

One day when Zechariah's section of priests was on duty, he was the one chosen to enter the sanctuary to offer incense to the Lord. This was a task Zechariah had performed many times in the past, but this time things went differently than usual. While Zechariah was praying in the sanctuary, an angel of the Lord appeared to him to tell him that his prayers had been heard; his wife was finally going to have a child, and they were to name the child John. John would be great in the eyes of the Lord and would turn the children of Israel back to God.

No doubt, Zechariah had spent years praying for and envisioning the day when he would learn that his prayers, and those of Elizabeth, were finally answered. No doubt he had imagined how that day would play out. He had probably imagined feeling joy as he shared the news with his family members and friends. He had probably imagined his wonder as his wife's body started to change to accommodate the new life growing within her. He probably imagined that he would praise God in a loud voice as the shame was lifted from his family. But in that moment in the sanctuary, Zechariah was completely caught off-guard by the news. In that moment, his biggest feeling was doubt. He was in complete disbelief that this could really be happening. How could he go home and tell his wife that their troubles were over because she was pregnant? And so, he spoke the only words he could muster: "How will I know this is so?" He even offered the excuse of his age and his wife's age as rationales as to why he asked such a question. And as punishment for his doubt, Zechariah was rendered mute until the day the child was born.

This family could not seem to catch a break. For all their righteousness, this family just could not seem to escape their public shame. Elizabeth was now enduring the public shame of enduring a pregnancy beyond her natural childbearing years. She was out of place. She would not have fit in with the teens and twenty-somethings around town. She would officially be shunned by her fellow thirty and forty-somethings who already had adult children, and probably even grandchildren. And to top things off, she had a husband who didn't say a word! The man who usually whispered words of encouragement into her ear could only offer her a longing glance to comfort her fears. The man who would have been the one to speak out on her behalf in the public square could only give a stern look to the folks who whispered about her. A moment that should have been filled with celebration became a bit of a personal crisis.

The good news of the crisis is that Elizabeth could be of assistance to another woman who was dealing with a pregnancy at the most inconvenient of times. When I think about this newfound relationship Elizabeth and Mary formed out of their mutually inconvenient circumstances, I call to mind the story of Esther, the Jewish girl who became a Persian queen because of the rather inconvenient disposal of the former queen. Esther's position as queen was precarious because it was clear that she was now married to a king with a short fuse for any disagreement from his queens. When her cousin, Mordecai, learned of the plans to carry out a mass genocide of their people, he wrote to her saying that perhaps she was on the throne "for such a time as this" (Esther 4:14). Now, there are many social problems in the book of Esther. First, I notice the king's choice to banish Vasthi for refusing to dance naked before him and his drunken male guests. Second, I notice the choice to bring the king virgins from throughout the empire to entertain him. One of those young women, without her consent, would be chosen to replace Vasthi on the throne. Third, I notice the king's disregard of the actions of one of his senior leaders, Haman, who threatened to carry out an action that would harm the queen's people, and perhaps even the queen herself. But I also notice the grace in the story. Had Vasthi never been banished and had Esther never become queen, the children of Israel would have been systematically exterminated without a second thought. Esther and Elizabeth both endured shame that was unjust. They both endured trauma to their bodies they never should have endured. However, they also learned, and they teach us, what grace looks like. Our inconvenient and uncomfortable circumstances are an opportunity to be a supporter of other people. It is the amazing grace of God that turns shame into triumph.

Elizabeth's shame became her greatest triumph. When she learned that she was pregnant, she went into seclusion for five months and said of her condition in Luke 1:25, "This is what the Lord has done for me when he looked favorably on me and took away the disgrace I have endured among my people." Because of where Elizabeth had been, she had a greater appreciation for the new life developing within her. We do not know what she knew about her child's future. Zechariah had received prophetic words about who their child would be but had not been able to share the news with Elizabeth because he was rendered mute. She did not love this new life growing inside of her because of who he would become. She loved this new life because he would be. She, as an older mother, surrendered her body. Unlike many of the women who had older female mentors as their bodies changed to accommodate new life, she had no wise sisters to call upon. She only had herself and her unrelenting faith in and devotion to God.

Elizabeth had her faith, but she still needed her sisterhood. In the first chapter, we talked about Eve and the loneliness she must have felt as she was the first woman to ever bring new life into the world. She would not have known what to expect. She would not have known what was taking place in her body. She, for all her desire to eat from the tree of the knowledge of good and evil would have been taught by her body that she knew nothing. We have all, in a moment of utter humility, come to that conclusion in the past, or if we continue to live in these fallible bodies we will one day. I think of all my dear, accomplished, wise, well-educated, generous, kind, and loving friends who despite their efforts to live on the "right" path have found themselves battling diseases (both mental and physical) that are beyond their control. Those are moments when we realize that no amount of education, good humor, or generosity of spirit mean that we have any amount of the knowledge of good and evil. The moments that it seems that our bodies fail us cause us to understand that we only see the totality of good and evil in part. Our own humanity obscures our vision. These broken vessels of clay we inhabit are holy, but that does not make them any less broken. It is our arduous task to discover the holiness in that which is broken rather than allowing our brokenness to force us into seclusion.

I am amazed by Elizabeth's story because she takes the pregnancy news in stride, and even praises God for blessing her with something so beautiful that has taken away her shame. She says she is not ashamed and that she believes God favors her, but based on her actions, I do not quite believe her. I imagine that she might have ventured out from time to time to get necessities from the market, but as soon as her pregnancy became apparent to the people around her, she refused to leave the house. Her blessing was too much for her, and the shame she had carried for her entire adult life quickly returned to her. I make this observation about Elizabeth uncritically. In fact, I think it is a reaction that many of us find relatable. Women face critiques, both from within ourselves and from the world, each time our bodies change. For example, women who lose significant amounts of weight often feel ashamed post weight loss because of the excess skin on their bodies, the misguided "congratulatory" comments, and the pile of clothes that no longer fit. Likewise, women whose bodies are recovering from illnesses often feel shame as their bodies return to the new version of good health. Girls often feel shame as our bodies develop through our adolescent years. No doubt, to this day, women who become mothers in their thirties and forties like Elizabeth did feel shame because of the changes happening in their bodies. Many women over fifty feel ashamed as their bodies change during menopause. We carry a lot of shame about our bodies. Elizabeth's reaction to her presence mirrors the reaction that many of us have had to changes in our bodies.

The good news is, we are never experiencing chaos alone. As Renita Weems puts it in her book *Showing Mary: How Women Can Share Prayers, Wisdom, and The Blessings of God,* "Elizabeth's pregnancy shows that no matter how unbelievable your situation seems, no matter how unfathomable it all sounds, another woman somewhere is experiencing her own share of holy chaos as she stands by, just like you are, watching her life come undone." Weems goes on to explain that it was no coincidence that Mary and Elizabeth ended up pregnant at the same time. In the final chapter of this book, which is about Mary, I focus on the importance of adult women teaching teenage women the value in their bodies. But what we notice if we look at the relationship between Mary and Elizabeth differently is Elizabeth's humility when encountered with a teenage mother. Elizabeth accepted sisterhood from a woman who had significantly less life experience than she did. She could recognize holiness when it approached her. This text calls us to value sacred sisterhoods across generational lines. Meanwhile, we must celebrate Mary, who could have gone to any number of teenage friends to receive guidance about her circumstances, but she chose her cousin. She knew that God was doing something special in her life when in Luke 1:36 the angel of the Lord tells her of Elizabeth's pregnancy. The testimony of God's incredible work in another woman's life showed Mary that anything was also possible in her life.

Mary's visit with Elizabeth lasted about three months. What bonds of sacred sisterhood were forged during that time? I imagine that Elizabeth finally felt empowered to go out. These two would have made an odd pair as they traveled around town together—two women who should have (according to societal standards) been ashamed of their conditions but instead walked with confidence because they knew that God was doing something incredible through their bodies. And the time came, and Elizabeth gave birth. Luke 1:58 tells us that Elizabeth's friends and relatives came to see her because they heard that the Lord had shown great mercy to her. But on the contrary, I would argue that Elizabeth bore great mercy into the world. Through her sacred sisterhood with Mary that brought them both into a deeper understanding of the ways of God, through her courage amidst extreme change, and through her acceptance of God's holy timing, Elizabeth was the living embodiment of the great mercy of God as she birthed one of the greatest prophets of scripture. Her body bore great mercy.

Prayer: Dear Lord, I declare that I will not harbor shame over the changes that are happening inside me. Maybe my life is changing for such a time as this. Help me to seek out sacred friendships that will empower me to walk in the promise You have placed on my life. I do not always understand Your timing, yet I thank You for the new things You are doing within me. Amen.

CHAPTER 4

THERE WAS ALSO A PROPHET, ANNA: LUKE 2:36–38

*M*y mother is amazing. From the moment she first knew I was in her womb, she nurtured me. Already a woman in peak physical condition at the time, she worked even harder during her pregnancy to take good care of her body. She continued to exercise passionately, she ate the healthiest food available, and with my father, she prepared to welcome a new life into the world. As a military couple living an ocean away from their families, they surrounded themselves with a community of caring friends who prepared alongside them for my arrival. I know the abiding love of these friends from almost three decades ago because some of reach out to me using social media. They earnestly attempt to reconnect with my parents and to let me know that although I don't remember ever having met them, they care about me and are eager to partner with me on my current journey.

My mother still talks about giving birth to me. Do all mothers do that? She remembers that I arrived about a week after my due date, how broad my shoulders were, and that I was a quiet baby. When she called my godmother to let her know that I had been born, my godmother didn't believe it because she didn't hear the cries of a newborn baby. I was born in Germany, where both of my parents were stationed at the time, so my mother also remembers the struggle to find clothes that would fit me properly since German newborns were stockier than I was! Although I was small, she recalls that I was strong and had a voracious appetite. The other babies would slowly drink their bottles and had to be goaded to drink everything. I drank my bottles quickly and hungrily and then had no trouble drifting off to sleep. My mother also remembers being teased by her family and friends because in my early years, I looked just like my father. She recalls that she was often described as the "human incubator." The memory of me bearing so little resemblance to my mother is ironic now because we look so much alike today.

In my school years, my mother continued to nurture me. She taught me to exercise, packed nutritious lunches (that I did not always eat), and most of all, I credit my mother with teaching me to have a strong work ethic. She insisted that I begin taking piano lessons at age four; I remember awakening at the crack of dawn throughout my adolescence to practice for an hour before school. She demanded excellence on all my school work, she supported me in my dance training, she cheered me on as a cross country runner, she affirmed my intellect, and she encouraged me to dream big. Like many other mother-daughter pairs, our relationship has never been perfect.

We have disagreed about everything from wardrobe to hair to diet to professional decisions. But our longest standing disagreement has surrounded the question of who I am meant to be. As an only child, I have found myself under pressure that I think is best understood by other only children and eldest children. Our parents' hopes and dreams are centered on us becoming the people they believe they brought us into this world to be. For me, my mother's dreams for me as I understand them were that I would be a woman of strong faith and moral conviction, that I would be healthy from the inside out, and that I would be a high achiever professionally, personally, and academically.

When I was growing up, I often misunderstood my mother's dreams for me. I thought she wanted me to be perfect, and since I will never be perfect, the pressure infuriated me. It was clear to me that I would always fall short. During much of my adolescence, I thought she could not have cared less about the woman I wanted to be. My mother and I still have setbacks in our relationship. We always will, because human relationships are challenging and dynamic. The good news is that we are also both growing in love and maturing. We are learning how to care for one another. As I grow in love and maturity, I am also coming to better understand how much she loves me. I am learning to honor the prayers and hopes and dreams she has for me. At my core, I am beginning to share her dreams for me. I want to be faithful to God and humanity because God loves me so well. I want to be healthy because I owe myself and God a basic level of self-care. I will strive to be a high achiever in all that I do to honor my Creator, my ancestors, my family members, and my friends who have sacrificed so much so that I could thrive. Although my parents enforced strict discipline during my youth, I think the dreams they had and still have for me mirror the dreams that many parents have for their children. Most parents dream that their children will become happy, healthy, and productive adults, but they do not always know how to relate those dreams to their children.

As I work on this book, I see that the tensions my mother and I have had with one another in our relationship have existed between parents and their children since the beginning of human history as found in the Bible. Parents have been reluctant to connect with their children as fully formed beings with genuine opinions. Meanwhile, children have been reluctant to heed a parent's wisdom, preferring to rely on knowledge gained outside of the families of origin. And the tension, specifically the tension that exists between mothers and their offspring, is probably because mothers are cocreators with God. The seeds of life are planted and grow inside them. They feel they understand the intention with which their children came to be. That maternal self-assuredness inspired the interventionist actions of Rebekah that we talked about in chapter 2.

I have enduring respect for women who have physically birthed children. But I want to take the next two chapters to hold space for two New Testament women whose bodies bore the Word without them ever physically giving birth because, as I stated in the introduction, female bodies matter. In the next two chapters, I interrogate the work of the female body that lives and dies without producing offspring. I have spent so much time on the last few pages discussing my relationship with my biological parents because our biological parents, or whoever took on primary responsibility for raising us, shape our lives in distinct ways. Yet our lives are also distinctly shaped by a series of women we meet throughout our lives who, whether they have ever borne children of their own or not, shape us, mother us, nurture us, and inspire the best in us.

I want to take some time to examine what it is to be a woman whose body is in shape to be used by God, but who never physically carries a child in her womb, for, as I expressed in the introduction, women's bodies are worthwhile. We needn't carry children in our wombs to justify our womanhood. A woman is she who wakes up each morning and chooses to live into her womanhood. As you read these chapters, hold in your heart a woman who you know (perhaps you are that woman) who because of physical or social challenges will never bear children or who is beyond childbearing years and has never had a child. I have three such women in my heart as I write. I have known these women at different stages of my life, and all three of them have been surrogate mothers to me. They haven't stepped into that mother role because my biological mother was lacking in any way, for, as I have stated in the preceding paragraphs, my mother is extraordinary. No, these women have mothered me because they felt led by the Holy Spirit to sow into the life of a young woman whom they believed was interesting, creative, intelligent, curious, and promising. I do not know whether I will ever bear children of my own, but these women are a reminder to me that my womanhood, my ability to call myself a mother, and my ability to inspire future generations of young women is not bound up in the capabilities of my reproductive system. My body can and will bear the Word. Their bodies can and do bear the Word for me.

As I write these words, I recall the words written by an evangelical theologian, preacher, and blogger named Jory Micah. In July of 2016, Micah published a blog post entitled "I Am a Woman." In the honest post, Micah explains that despite her brokenness and flaws, her womanhood does not place limits on her giftedness or her call. She explains that she struggles with anxiety. She is anxious about whether her marriage will last, when or how she will become a mother, what her next career steps should be, and whether she will regain weight she has lost. She admits that she is even anxious about being anxious. The reason my mind returns to this post is because it so beautifully encapsulates what it is to be a Christian woman. We want to live into our spiritual gifts which have been sown in our souls by our congregations and our Creator, yet there are roadblocks and restrictions at every turn. We want to be in healthy relationships and mother families of our own, but we also understand that no amount of faith guarantees an outwardly perfect life. We want clear roadmaps about our careers, but we also understand that there is a time to wait on God to order our steps. We understand that our bodies are temples and we want to honor them, but we struggle with our overall health. We fight against our flesh daily it seems. Why? Because we are women. We struggle because we are here.

The beautiful part of it all is that the holy struggle is what this life of faith is all about. The less-than-beautiful part is that knowing that this holy struggle is part of the faithful life does not make the struggle less painful. Perhaps the most challenging part of womanhood is the performative nature of gender identity. Despite the pain that so many women endure within our bodies and outside of them because of our womanhood, we are told to be beautiful in the ways the world has defined beauty. The sexist standard extends even into our churches where, although we are taught that God created us fearfully and wonderfully, we are also told very specific ways we ought to present our bodies. Sometimes we are given this body advice because of concern about modesty. But I have found more often than not that we are given unsolicited advice to help us attract or "keep" a mate. There seems to be no consideration of the idea that perhaps instead of forcing ourselves into carbon copies of one notion of what it is to be a beautiful Christian woman, we could live instead more fully into the natural beauty God placed on that planet when God created each of us.

The woman who is the subject of this chapter probably endured significant pain throughout her life. We meet our prophet friend Anna when Jesus was only about forty days old. The laws of the Hebrew Bible demanded that every firstborn male had to be set aside as holy to the Lord. So, Joseph and Mary made the trip to the temple in Jerusalem to present Jesus and to make a sacrifice of two pigeons. Their gesture was common. Many faithful Jewish couples would have carried out the ritual every day, so they should not have stood out for this ordinary act of piety. They stood out to those who had eyes to see not because of their act but because of the child who was involved in the act. This was a presentation of the Messiah in Jerusalem. Most of the people in Jerusalem would not have noticed the trio as they traveled through the city. The Israelites had been waiting for the Messiah for centuries. The Messiah was expected to be a great king who would deliver Israel from the hands of her enemies. But that is not who Jesus was. He was easy to miss. Jesus wore street clothes, so if He walked down the streets of our neighborhoods, many of us would miss Him too.

But not everyone mistook Joseph, Mary, and Jesus for one of Israel's ordinary young families. Two faithful old Israelites knew exactly who these folks were. The first of these actors, Simeon, usually gets quite a bit of attention. His words of praise to God in Luke 2:29–32 are, "Master, now you are dismissing your servant in peace, according to your word; for my eyes have seen your salvation, which you have prepared in the presence of all peoples, a light for revelation to the Gentiles and for glory to your people Israel." His prayer is today called the "Nunc Dimittis." If you are the type of person who likes to attend church during the Christmas season, you have no doubt heard a sermon or two about Simeon's great faith. It had been revealed to him earlier in his life that he would not die until he saw the Messiah. So, on the day that Jesus's parents brought Him to the temple, Simeon was guided by the Spirit to be there as well. As soon as Simeon saw the family, he took the child into his arms to praise God and turned to his astounded (and no doubt slightly fearful) mother to prophesy about who

Jesus would become and to warn her of the inevitable pain she was to endure as Jesus's mother.

Much has been made of Simeon's prophetic words in our theological renderings of the life and meaning of Jesus. Meanwhile, Anna, who appears in the same story doing something even more astounding with her body and her time, becomes a footnote in this pivotal story of how Israel was first introduced to her Messiah. But of the two, Anna is the one who Luke describes as a "prophet." In his book, *Strong Was Her Faith: Women of the New Testament*, J. Ellsworth Kalas says of Anna that she "is the first person named a prophet in the New Testament. She was a generation ahead of John; but in a quiet way she had the same calling, to prepare the way for the Messiah."

On the day that Jesus came to the temple, Simeon was compelled by the Spirit to go there too. But Anna. Anna was different. Anna never left the temple. Of course, we are not meant to take such a statement literally since every function of life could not have happened in the temple. But we all know those women (and certain men) who spend much of their lives improving their community of faith in some way, although they are never called religious leaders within the community. These individuals exercise a particular kind of discipline over their minds, bodies, and spirits that is remarkable. We know instinctively that they must eat, drink, sleep, and use the facilities, but we are not sure when they tend to themselves. They are compelled by love to be where they feel God has called them to be. In my pastoral experience, I notice that these folks are often unappreciated and unseen, but the shape they keep their minds, bodies, and spirits in, and our religious communities, as a result, should not be taken for granted. This incredible prophet, Anna, only gets a few verses in scripture, but she had the all-important role of letting the people of Jerusalem know that the Messiah had finally arrived. They did not have to live in darkness anymore.

Anna didn't have a traveling ministry. She was not the rabbi whom everyone sought out for advice. Anna was a fixture in the temple. I imagine that she didn't say much to anyone. I imagine that she didn't draw too much attention to herself. Aside from her prophetic status, Anna was an afterthought even in her own world. She had been married for seven years and then widowed. Her life was challenging, yet Anna only focused on obedience to God. She knew that if she stayed in the temple and worshiped, day and night, a change would come, and come, it did.

You see, Anna is a reminder to those of us for whom things just don't seem to happen the way that we might want them too that if we stay plugged into the life of the Spirit day and night, something is going to happen. Scripture promises us continually that God has plans for us and that God's plan for us is that we prosper. Anna is a reminder to somebody that if you believe you are in God and you are not prospering yet, God has a plan; find a Sanctuary to which you feel called, and start doing some holy waiting. As a notoriously impatient person, a call to holy waiting troubles me. I often tell people that my favorite thing about fast food is that it is fast. The trick to waiting is to understand that we have a job while we wait—that is, to prepare. In other words, work while you wait. People who wait on God are never really just waiting. They are preparing the way in the wilderness.

Be open to the possibility that God has something great in store for you that you might never imagine. Be confident in the assurance that God might not perform this great thing in your life in the timing you expect but that it will happen. Anna, at eighty-four years old, was far beyond her childbearing years on the day that Jesus was brought into the temple by Joseph and Mary, but her worship bore that holy child.

Kalas explains in his further discussion of Anna that the Catholic tradition continued her story, even teaching lessons such as Anna becoming a tutor to young Mary as she matured on her faith journey. These stories are beautiful but have no basis in scripture. The story we find in Luke 2:36–38 is more than enough. Women joined Jesus on His journey to Calvary in many ways. Although Mary was the only one to physically birth Him, others manipulated their bodies, minds, and spirits to accommodate Him. The first of these women were Elizabeth and Anna. It seems that history has an unspoken rule that women, if they are to be included in history, must perform superhuman acts. But women like Anna demonstrate that holy waiting and profound faith are superhuman acts. Our mothers are the women who see us, even as young children, and speak life to us. Our mothers are the ones who celebrate us for no other reason than because we exist. Our mothers are the ones who are willing to wait for us.

Prayer: Lord, I am waiting. I am in pain because of all my waiting. Grant me the holy perseverance to continue to wait and trust You to show me the calling You have placed on my life. When I have found that call, help me, like Anna, to go out, sharing my gift with the world. With all that I am, I desire to bear Your Word to the world. Amen.

CHAPTER 5

MARY'S HAIR SHARED HER TESTIMONY JOHN 12:1–8

As women, we are often hair obsessed. It sometimes feels as though we are fully known by the world based on their perception of a single strand of our hair. I have had riveting conversations with women of all races and cultures about how they were taught to think about their hair, what their mother said about their hair, how long it takes for them to tame their hair before leaving the house, and the comments others have made to them about their hair. There are countless videos on the Internet featuring women with coarse or curly hair textures speaking about the challenges of their hair. As women, how we wear our hair matters. Many of us have close friends or family members (or we ourselves) who have struggled through treatment for cancer and have lost hair. Many women have been taught that our hair is our beauty and to cut our hair (and certainly to be bald) is to somehow diminish or to completely destroy our beauty.

The things we hear about hair subconsciously reinforce the idea that our hair holds greater value than our lives.

The dialogue about hair is even more intense among women black and brown women. I have heard many a Latina woman declare that her family was concerned when she got a short haircut, as though her femininity were bound in her hair. Many black women have felt the sting of hearing that our "natural" hair is somehow inappropriate to be worn in professional or academic settings. We are being told that what God placed on our heads was someone wrong or damaged. Within our own communities, we critique one another regularly for the hair choices we make. Every woman's defenses are high to explain why she wears her hair the way that she does. These debates are so frequent that singer-songwriter India Arie released a song in 2006 called "I Am Not My Hair." In the chorus of the song, Arie sings, "I am not my hair, I am not this skin, I am not your expectations, no, no. I am not my hair, I am not this skin, I am a soul that lives within."

And then there are the conversations about what we ought (and ought not) do with our hair and the hair of others in public. Women and girls are often critiqued for all the places our hair ends up. Women's hair can be found in drains, stuck to clothes, and attached to bags. Although shedding hair is completely natural, we can be hard on each other. We seem to say to each other in our critiques, "How hard is it to keep your hair on your head?" And then, there is the hair touching. My tidbit of friendly advice for all of us is to keep our hands off each other's heads. But there seems to be this temptation held by so many of us to touch each other's hair. Disproportionately, black and brown women must endure having perfect strangers either ask to touch our hair or simply placing their hands in our scalps without so much as an oral greeting. In her 2016 song, "Don't Touch My Hair," Solange Knowles sings the lyrics that rest on the hearts of so many women, "Don't touch my hair, When it's the feelings I wear, Don't touch my soul, When it's the rhythm I know, Don't touch my crown, They say the vision I've found. Don't touch what's there, When it's the feelings I wear." We hold so much passion in our hair, and in the lack thereof. Whether we appreciate it or not, women's hair matter. Many of us, for better or for worse, have soul connections with our hair.

Jesus had a soul connection with a certain family who lived in Bethany, just east of Jerusalem. Mary, Martha, and their brother Lazarus often played host to Jesus. They shared meals together, but more than that, it was clear that Jesus had a bond of friendship love with them. Their relationship with Jesus was as personal as it gets. In John 11, Jesus performed the miraculous for this family by raising Lazarus when he had been dead for four days. The Jewish custom at that time required that burial happen on the day of the death, if possible. It also held that the soul lingered near the body for three days. Death was truly final on the fourth day, which made this miracle of Jesus even more miraculous and made Pharisee leadership despise Him even more (*HarperCollins Study Bible*, 1836–1837). This family invited Jesus to dine with them six days before the Passover, and as usual, they did something extravagant in the presence of Jesus. Martha served, Lazarus shared the table, and Mary took a pound of costly perfume, used it to anoint Jesus's feet, and wiped His feet with her hair. There is a similar story of a "sinful woman" who performed such an act of extravagant love in Mark 14:3–9, Matthew 26:6–13, and Luke 7:37–38, but only in the Gospel of John is the woman identified to be Mary, sister of Martha and Lazarus.

The Gospel of John relies on allegories to give us clues into the person of Jesus Christ. In this gospel, we find our most highly Christological Jesus. Jesus speaks in metaphors, most famously John 3's admonition to Nicodemus that to be saved one must be "born again." We as the contemporary believers ask the same question Nicodemus did that night, "How can anyone be born after having grown old?" It is also in this gospel that we meet the Samaritan woman at the well. Through her story, we learn that Jesus provides "living water." We as contemporary believers ask, as she did, "Where do you get that living water?" As J. Ellsworth Kalas points out in his book, *Strong Was Her Faith: Women of the New Testament*, "John's Gospel is marked by the author's use of double meanings."

John explains in John 12:3 that the entire house was filled with the fragrance of the perfume. Kalas explains that some of the early Christian theologians understood this to mean that the whole body of the church experienced the fragrance of Mary's deed. Mary's love was for Jesus was extravagant, unforgettable, and powerful. It was the kind of show of love that no one could ignore or deny. But immediately after her act, the people who witnessed it tried to diminish its value, critiquing her for being too extravagant and emotional. Judas Iscariot, the man who was soon to betray Jesus, asked why she had not sold the perfume instead and given the money to the poor. John clarifies Judas's critique by writing parenthetically that Judas was, in reality, a thief who did not care about the poor. And isn't that just the way things work when we put all that we have and all that we are on the line to love Jesus? Our most outspoken critics are the ones who have no conception of what it is to love. Their critiques are ironic, yet they shame us. They make us diminish ourselves. They cause us to question our motives. What I love about the way this story is told in all the Gospels is that Jesus defends Mary. In John, Jesus tells the room that she should be left alone because she bought to perfume "for the day of [His] burial." However, I love even more what Jesus says in Matthew 26 in this extravagantly loving woman's defense, "Truly I tell you, wherever this good news is proclaimed in the whole world, what she has done will be told in remembrance of her." Jesus, at that moment, moved her from being perceived as an overly emotional woman to being seen as a prophet and theologian with unique insight into Jesus's relevance to the human story. It is essential for us to understand and remember her story for us to comprehend Jesus's salvific work.

We encounter Mary (and her sister Martha) throughout the Gospels. They were women who maintained a close and meaningful friendship with Jesus. They were women and yet, their lives were defined by their actions vis-a-vi Jesus, not by their childbearing. And yet, their bodies bore the Word. They are yet another reminder that women's power is deeper than our reproductive capacity. We have minds, spirits, and indeed whole bodies that are worthy of being deployed in service to God.

Who can forget Martha's day laboring to serve Jesus recounted in Luke 10:38–42? Martha spent the day working in the kitchen without any help from the rest of her family because she believed that Jesus needed her to perform the domestic tasks of presenting a clean home and serving a meal. In all her haste and anxiety, she snapped. She could not ascertain why her sister spent the day sitting at Jesus's feet while she did all the housework. She demanded that Jesus compel her sister to be helpful, but Jesus said to her, "Martha, Martha, you are worried and upset about many things, but few things are needed." Through her misdirected domestic labor, Martha bore an essential lesson to us—that is that we are called to keep our minds, bodies, and spirits focused on the one thing to which we are called. Secondarily, she is a reminder to so many of us who believe that our busyness is a sign of our holiness that maybe that is a notion that it is time for us to rethink.

And then there is Mary. In contrast to her sister, Mary had an almost obsessive focus on Jesus. While Martha labored incessantly in the Luke 10 passage I just referenced, Mary sat the entire day at Jesus's feet listening to Him. I imagine that she neglected almost every physical need during that time, soaking in like a sponge each utterance that proceeded from Jesus's lips. Her stillness that day is a reminder to us that our bodies, minds, and spirits can find stillness in the presence of Jesus. Then there is the message of her hair, which is recounted elegantly in all of the four Gospels. My mind returns incessantly to the lyrics of India Arie and Solange Knowles, both of whom understand their hair to have soul relevance. In John 13:1–17, Jesus washes His disciples' feet which was an act of extreme humility that a servant might perform for his or her master. It was an action that ashamed the disciples because they understood Jesus to be of greater importance than them.

There is something shameful about our feet, isn't there? We rely heavily on our feet, and of course, in the setting of the Bible, many people would have had feet soiled by dirt and sand from long walks in the desert sands. But here was Mary, not a servant but a friend, who modeled the kind of love that Jesus demands of His followers. She entered the room with her most costly perfume and poured it upon the feet of Jesus. As though that act of humility and love were insufficient, Mary then proceeded to finish cleaning Jesus's feet with her hair. Some might say that this action was extravagant, but when we think about it, was it enough? Jesus, the divine, sacrificed His life for the sins of the world, and there is nothing we can do to repay that gift, but Mary brings us several steps closer to bridging that gap.

Mary (and her sister Martha) both present us with ways we may use our bodies to bear the Word into the world. They both represent the deeper power of women. They are also a reminder of Jesus's love for women. Jesus considered women to be friends and colleagues in ministry. Indeed, His relationship with Mary was so profound that she was the first to carry the good news of the resurrection into the world. Her body bore the Word.

Prayer: Dear Lord, thank You for the stories that I bear in my hair (or my lack thereof). May I use the fullness of my body in service to You. May I prophetically live out my deep and abiding love for You. May I be extravagant and fearless because You are worthy of all that I have because all that I have belongs to You. Amen.

CHAPTER 6

A VIRGIN'S LIFE: LUKE 1:26–38

I was never the best science student, but I did extremely well in ninth-grade biology. I did so well, in fact, that I can tell you that it is not every day that virgins conceive children. In fact, I can definitively tell you that it is not scientifically possible for a virgin to naturally conceive a child. Have you ever seen the television show *Jane the Virgin*? The show is a comedic telenovela that follows a Miami twenty-something named Jane, a student and aspiring writer, whose grandmother taught her to preserve her virginity until she was married. Jane faithfully kept her promise to her grandmother to maintain her virginity until she was married. One morning Jane goes to the gynecologist's office, and a substitute doctor accidentally artificially inseminates her. Jane conceives, and the show follows her as she tries to maintain her relationship with her fiancé, tries to build a relationship with the baby's father (and his wife), and attempts to balance her education, work, and life as a new mother.

If the show were not comedic, it would be far too exhausting to watch. The show is, of course, loosely playing with the themes of the story of the Virgin Mary. What happens when a young virgin conceives and bears a child? Chaos, that's what! It is the sort of situation that no one could prepare themselves to handle. The virginal body cannot become pregnant. Suddenly, the virgin and her family are forced to adjust their entire social dynamic. She feels pressure to maintain a committed relationship with a partner for the good of her child, and her body changes forever. What do we as the "mature ones" do with a young virgin who is suddenly rendered mature by the child in her womb?

Before I proceed, let's talk about this category of "virgin." The teachings of the church through the ages have told us that Mary conceived a child without sexual relations. There is no reason to discard that narrative. However, that narrative is also not a license to critique women for having (and perhaps daring to enjoy) sexual relations with a partner as somehow being less holy than Mary. Mary's story is not necessarily a critique of sex. In chapter 1, we discussed the entrance of sin into the world through the generations through childbirth. Since Jesus is sinless, God needed to find a way around that problem, so God decided to spiritually inseminate Mary.

While we traditionally think of a virgin as one who has had no sexual experience, I would posit to you that it might be helpful for us to recast a virgin as one who chooses purity in her life, regardless of her sexual experiences or lack thereof. In her devotional book, *Showing Mary: How Women Can Share Prayers, Wisdom, and the Blessings of God*, biblical scholar Renita Weems explains that in ancient times, the word *virgin* referred not to a physical state but instead to a woman's psychological attitude. A virgin, Weems explains, was "a woman who was still in touch with her own inner values and acted according to what she believed was true." So, a married woman who had sexual relations with her husband could have still been designated a virgin if she was true to herself. The virgin is the woman who lives in the world, and loves the world, but remains true to God and to herself. This is great news because it means that all of us can be the virgin, physically, emotionally, and spiritually.

Although that reframing of the term is useful, as a young, unmarried woman, and according to all indications in the text, I think we are meant to understand Mary's virginity at the time of Gabriel's visit according to the more traditional definition of the term. I imagine that Mary felt unprepared to take on the physical, emotional, mental, social, and spiritual burden of carrying a child. No doubt, she felt even more daunted as she came to terms with the fact that this child was the long-awaited Messiah. She probably developed a case of imposter's syndrome.

Many of us deal with imposter's syndrome. Imposter's syndrome is the distinct feeling that you are not meant to be where you currently find yourself. You feel like you have not earned the job, position, or status you currently have because everyone around you seems to have greater competency. This is a syndrome that women have disproportionately to men, and as a black woman, I find that my hyperqualified and intelligent sisters of color often deal with this syndrome in our personal and professional lives, no matter how confidently we carry ourselves. I have struggled with imposter's syndrome since my first semester of college, the idea that I was where I was because of some unprecedented mistake. As I mentioned in my introduction, I attended a women's college, and many of my classmates expressed similar concerns. My intelligent, creative, and passionate sisters and I were floating in a pool of fear. It is no way to live.

Today, I am a woman called and set apart by God, qualified by my experience and training, and yet, on so many days, I feel underqualified and underprepared for what I know I can and should be doing. The feeling is frustrating because as people of faith, we know that God has already won the victory on our behalf! Despite that knowledge, so often we find ourselves fearing the rejection of other people. One Friday, I was at the end of a challenging week in ministry. I felt like I was fighting to defend my ministry. This fight happens on multiple fronts. In the twenty-first century, the face of the church is entirely different than it was even twenty or twenty-five years ago. A quarter century ago, strong seminary training and gifts and skills for professional ministry almost guaranteed a position as a minister at a church. Ministry no longer takes such straightforward paths for the majority of seminary graduates. Today's seminary graduate faces the task of determining what it looks like to do ministry in the world, whether that be in health care settings or schools or corporate environments or nonprofit organizations or something completely new and innovative. Many of us are forging our own paths. The wide-open nature of my field is both a discouragement and a motivator. It is discouraging in that there are no guarantees, but it is a motivator in that it presents the

Spirit-filled minister with an extraordinary opportunity to birth a new thing. It is almost like we have returned to the first-century church. It is our task to decide what the church will be.

But the decline of participation in mainline Protestant Churches is not the only thing that makes contemporary ministry a fight. As a young woman of color in ordained ministry, the battle happens daily. However, there are times when that battle feels more palpable than it does at other times. That week was one of those times. I felt overburdened, abused, and degraded, all because I wanted to carry out what I believed God was calling me to do. What frustrated me at the time was that I was carrying out my work in a church, not in a hospital or a school or a government institution, where I expected to be forced to defend the need for ministry.

While churches all over the world are challenged by the job of having to be the church, I find that churches at bottom behave like institutions. Institutions have a way of undervaluing, demeaning, and abusing the women that serve within them. Institutions tend to care more about their own self-preservation and less about the self-preservation of the people within them. The idea is that people are replaceable, but the institution is not. This is the way institutions behave, and while churches are institutions, we are called to be institutions that reflect the kingdom of God on earth, not institutions that conform to the behavior of this world. In as much as we Christians try to distinguish ourselves from the world, we often conform by appropriating its systemic hatred instead of rebuking it and choosing another way.

The challenging week I am describing occurred during the season of Advent. Advent is my absolute favorite season of the liturgical year. As a Protestant Christian raised in the Baptist tradition, I do not take time during the church year to remember the feast days of saints and martyrs like some of other traditions within the Christian faith do, but I do concern myself with the larger flow of the church year. Many Baptists have little regard for a liturgical year. However, as scripture teaches us in Ecclesiastes 3, "For everything there is a season, and a time for every matter under heaven." Thus, I celebrate Advent as the beginning of my church year. Advent is the season from the last Sunday in November until Christmas Eve during which Christians prepare for the coming of Christ, the light of the world. Advent is my favorite time in the church year because I find the idea that God chose to send a child to redeem a flawed world to be so elegant. God sent a baby, born in a dirty stable, to redeem us. This child teaches us that youthful innocence is redemptive.

Young girls all over the world have portrayed Mary in church plays and pageants. When I was fourteen years old, I was asked to portray Mary in my church's production of the Christmas story. The show demanded a lot out of everyone involved. It was complete with my dress being stuffed with pillows to add the weight of pregnancy to my small teenage frame, spotlights to highlight key moments, and a grown man to play Joseph (just to keep things realistic). During the nativity scene portion of the play, I was to hold a rather unattractive baby doll and to look at it lovingly as though it were my newborn baby. I did not enjoy the role. During the fake pregnancy scene, I was too hot because of the spotlights and the extra pillow weight. Then I had to pretend to love a doll, and worst of all, I had to put myself in the frame of mind of a young girl who selflessly surrendered all she had because she wanted to do the will of God. She put her womb and her reputation on the line because an angel told her that God had chosen her. For the first time, I was forced to come face-to-face with the sheer wonder of it all.

I was sure I was nothing like Mary. She was a teenage girl who God had chosen to bring Jesus into the world through her womb, and she had boldly taken on the role, almost without question. But I had lots of questions! I just knew that as a teenager, I would never be ready to take on any such godly task that would so disrupt the path of my life. One of the church choir directors asked me one day before the show how I felt about playing Mary. I told her that I didn't like it. I felt that I could not relate to Mary because I could and would never do what Mary did. The choir director looked at me and told me that she thought I was a lot like Mary.

God has a sense of humor. A year later, when I was fifteen, I realized that I was called to Christian ministry. It is a call that never left me, and it is a call that has changed my life. While my circumstances are nowhere near the level of gravity of the ones Mary was under, Mary is godmother to each of us who has felt God tugging on our hearts to do a new thing for the kingdom, something we were unprepared to do, something we did not quite understand, something that seemed impossible and we chose to follow it anyhow, even knowing our lives would be forever changed. In my experience, without my consent, my life has become a spectacle for the cause of Christ. I have learned two things from my experience.

First, I have learned that God calls teenage girls to do the work of God in the world. To put a finer point on it, God can use even the humble, fearful, virginal teenage body to bring new life into a broken world. The Mary story should cause us to wonder what young teenage girls have to teach us if we are willing to listen. Second, I have learned that Mary's burden was hers and that our burdens are our own. The connection between Mary and us is that each of us has some burden that God has placed upon our lives. The word *burden* ordinarily has a negative connotation, but here, it is being used to describe any load that we carry because God has told us it is ours to carry. Often it turns out that these loads we understood to be burdens are gifts. I will explain in the coming paragraphs.

Back to my challenging week in ministry. While I think we can sometimes over-spiritualize practical issues, I do believe that when we are in moments of Spirit clarity, the devil loves to emerge in various ways to block, remove, or otherwise diminish that clarity. During the week in question, I was surrounded by petty, long-standing issues that were distractions from the work that God was calling me to do. The pettiness of the entire affair enraged me. My first task was to pray that God would help me to control my feelings of anger and to redirect those feelings into feelings that would benefit the kingdom of God. Anger is not a sin. Scripture teaches us that it is acceptable to be angry so long as our anger does not cause us to sin. In my experience with anger, my sustained anger over day-to-day things can only lead me to sin. So, I had to channel my anger so I could continue to do the work I was called to do in my congregational setting in ways that were healthy and fulfilling for all involved parties.

As the day came to an end at last, the scripture the Holy Spirit placed on my heart was, "For with God, nothing will be impossible." "For with God, nothing will be impossible." The verse was not a resolution for my current concerns. No, the verse resounded in my mind because it was God's encouragement to keep me focused on where I was going. One thing that is important for ministers to understand about our own work is that everything we do is only temporary. We are to be under-shepherds of God doing the work that God calls us to do in each season. We also must be attuned to the voice of the Spirit telling us that it is time to do a new thing. I liken this to the experience of Abram in the book of Genesis. God told Abram to gather his family and his things, to leave the place that he had lived for his entire life, and to go to the place that God would show him, and Abram went. Ministry is a lot like that. God does give us places to land along the way where we feel fulfilled and cared for, but the time always comes when God tells us that it is time to go. Sometimes God gives us a specific location to head toward, but in my experience, God often says, "Go to the place that I will show you." And for a type-A personality like mine, the ambiguous "go" elicits unshakable feelings of anxiety. I had to take a step back at the end of the challenging week to stop blaming systems I could not change and people I was not and to seriously look inside myself and to wonder what was going on with me. And what God said to me was, "Nothing will be impossible."

I simply could not stop that verse from repeating in my mind, almost on loop, as I anxiously thought about my work and my calling, so I went to find the scripture reference. And there it was, plain as day in Luke 1:37 at the end of Mary's encounter with the angel who told her that she would be the mother of the Son of the Most High. Mary did not know how this could be because of the virginal state of her body, but the angel told her that nothing would be impossible with God. In that moment, I was once again the teenage girl, afraid of her calling. I had to surrender again my entire mind, soul, and body to do the work of God, to bear the word made flesh into the world. I was reminded again that God can use my body. I can use my body to glorify God; I can use my body as a tool of transformation. I need this body to be in the kind of shape for God to use it. Getting our bodies in that kind of shape is about more than the physical. Having a body that is usable for God's purposes requires being a virgin in the way that Renita Weems reimagines it for us. It requires us to be the sort of people who are all in for God.

Now, as an adult woman, I know that I am one of the blessed ones. Even as a girl, the women around me affirmed my worth. They allowed me to speak for myself. They recognized the potential within me. When I fell short, they demanded better out of me. When I aimed higher, they taught me that I could do more than I thought I could. Yes, I was a child, but no woman who was allowed into my life treated me as though my age made me or my ideas trivial, and if an adult woman ever thought to trivialize me because of my age, my mother was my staunchest advocate.

Of course, my transition from adolescence to adulthood had its share of bumps and bruises, but I was never broken because I was taught as a girl that there was no end to my potential. I remember one woman in ministry giving me a birthday card when I turned twenty-two. She wrote inside the door that I should "kick the door in with my pumps." I was taught that there was no tension between my femininity and my strength. I was taught that I could be Christian and free. I was taught that I could be endlessly compassionate and yet love myself enough to say no to the things that were not for my good. My mind and my spirit were guarded during my formative years. As I noted in the introduction, I cannot say the same for my body. Sometimes we preserve the minds and spirits of teenage girls, and I am forever grateful to the adults who guarded my mind and spirit. It is rare to find the woman or girl, of any age, whose body has been guarded.

The story of Mary, this virginal girl, whose body began to do a new and unexpected thing, ought to remind adults of our responsibility to the changing adolescent female body in whatever form it takes. In chapter 3, I wrote about the way Elizabeth, as an older woman, honored the change in Mary's body. She did not question her, and she did not shame her. She accepted her. For three months, they shared a home and allowed their bodies to go through complex changes together. Can you imagine? Aging pregnant woman, sitting alongside young, virginal pregnant teenager, changing together. As adult women, we all know the shame that comes with residing in these female bodies. Our height is never quite right, and our weight is never quite right. We face judgment and ridicule because of whom we choose, or do not choose, to share our bodies with sexually. While I am not, and will never, endorse premarital sex among teenagers, I also will never endorse shaming teenage girls for their sexual decisions. So many teenage girls make rash decisions about how to handle their bodies sexually because adult women have failed them. We have a responsibility to our baby sisters to teach them to love themselves body, mind, and spirit. We have an obligation to treat girls as though their bodies matter. We owe it to our baby sisters to sit beside them, as Elizabeth did with her cousin Mary, loving them, celebrating them, and exploring the wonders of the changes within their bodies, and our own, as gifts from God.

Prayer: Dear Lord, I thank You because nothing is impossible with You! Teach me that my potential is boundless. Help me to link arms with my sisters, reminding them of the value of their bodies, minds, and intellect. Thank You for blessing me with this body fit for service to You! Amen.

CONCLUSION

WHAT WORD DOES
YOUR BODY BEAR?

From Eve to the Virgin Mary and beyond, these bodies that God has gifted us bear the Word in profound ways. As I have worked on this book, I have spent significant time examining my relationship to my body. This writing process has been a spiritual exercise for me in that it has led to two discoveries. First, it has led me to a deeper appreciation of both the limits and the possibilities of my body. Second, it has led me to concentrate less on the things I despise about my body and to focus more on how my body can be of service, or how it can be a God-bearer.

Regarding the limits of my body, during the production of this book, I have spent significant time exercising my body. For me, physical exercise has always been a time for me to connect with God in new and profound ways. When I run, bike, or hike, I pray. The problem for me has always been the issue of self-judgment. I wonder why I cannot run faster, or why my body becomes exhausted in too short a time, or why certain tasks I believe should be easy for my body to perform present challenges. Perhaps I am being too lax by using the words *I wonder*. In reality, I am a harsh critic of my body. I desire at once for my body to be long and lean like a top model or ballerina, but I also want the tough, quick, and sturdy body of a gymnast or sprinter. I reside in a constant state of frustration, and at times resentment, because my body is less than perfect. So, as I have written this work, I have also begun the process of appreciating my physical limitations. As I complete work on this manuscript, it is the season of Lent. During Lent, we remember Jesus's sojourn in the desert during which He fasted and prayed for forty days. How His body must have yearned for food! After overcoming the temptation of the devil, scripture says that angels came and waited on Jesus. We need to have enough hunger, enough limits, and enough lack that we can allow the angels to come and wait upon us. Yes, our bodies have limits, and yes, our bodies fail, and just there is where God steps in to make up the difference.

Then there are the possibilities of my body. As I wrote in the preceding paragraph, in the past several months, exercise has been a major priority for me. I have always been a fairly fit person, but I have also relearned that I can improve my body and my physical health. By no means do these improvements come overnight; often physical improvements are not even apparent over the course of a few months, but with patience, grace, and self-love, our bodies begin to change. As our bodies change, we become enlightened as to the possibilities of our bodies. It was what Eve experienced as the first child-bearer in human history. It was what Rebekah experienced as she overcame the pain of a difficult pregnancy. It was what Elizabeth experienced as she became a first-time mother when she was already beyond her childbearing years. It was what Anna experienced as she prayed in the temple every day expecting the Messiah. It was what Mary experienced as her hair became her witness. It was what a Virgin from Nazareth experienced when she learned of the new life stirring within her. Our bodies bear possibilities that are beyond our wildest dreams.

Your body can, and does, bear the Word into the world. The question then is, "What word does my body bear?" Your body matters, and it is doing essential work. How can your body aid you in transforming your world? How can you love yourself and your body and your God enough to use your body as a tool for liberation and transformation? The time is now for you to use your fearfully and wonderfully made body to bear good news and hope to the world. So, let's get to it!

DISCUSSION QUESTIONS

Introduction: How Can This Be: Giving Our Bodies a Theology

1. Welcome to this study of body love theology. What are you hoping to gain from this study?
2. How has your faith journey impacted your relationship to your body?
3. What would be different about you in your faith if valuing female bodies was an essential part of your theology?
4. During this study, what will you work with God to cocreate?

Chapter 1: Eve Bore Seth to Replace Abel: Genesis 4:25

1. Do you think it is possible for us to honor (or dishonor) God through our eating habits? Using a journal, create a dietary plan for yourself that reflects the relationship that you would like to have with God. Include what you might have for breakfast, lunch, and dinner and any snacks you might have between meals. How might your life

change if you and God worked out your personal nutrition plan and you chose to follow it?

2. In response to the great pain that must have been inflicted on her when Cain killed Abel and was banished, Eve bore another son. We have all faced serious disappointments in life. What is your most common response to significant setbacks or disappointments?

Chapter 2: Rebekah Bore Conflicted Nations: Genesis 25:21–28

1. We learn a lot from Rebekah's actions in Genesis 24 and 25. The first lesson she teaches us is about hospitality to strangers when she not only offers water to Isaac's servant but offers to water his camels too. Her hospitality was evidence that she was open to being part of the story of the formation of the nation of Israel. Her hospitality was a sign that God could use her. How can you show greater hospitality, even to those you have never met?

2. What is the relationship between intersectionality (a social science concept) and your Christian faith?

3. Rebekah felt an inner pain during her pregnancy that she probably struggled to explain to her friends, family, and neighbors. Have you ever felt a pain you could not quite understand? How do you work to overcome those pains?

4. Rebekah was comforted during her pregnancy after she understood the relationship between the children she was carrying. The problem then was

that she tried to intervene in their story. A lot of us try to help God with God's work. Have you ever done that? Do you think you can step back and allow God to be God?

Chapter 3: Elizabeth Bore Great Mercy: Luke 1:24–25 57–58

1. It is time to approach the imperfections of our bodies nonjudgmentally. What physical practices can you begin to adopt a nonjudgmental relationship with your body? Write down your ideas.

2. During Elizabeth's pregnancy, Zechariah was mute. One of the most critical needs in any relationship is effective communication. Write down all the ways (other than speaking) that you can communicate in your treasured relationships.

3. After reading this chapter, what inconvenient circumstances are you dealing with in your life that you now believe are happening so that you can provide grace to the people around you?

Chapter 4: There Was Also a Prophet, Anna: Luke 2:36–38

1. How did your immediate family nurture you during your childhood? Did they fail to nurture you in any way?

2. Are there any women who you would consider to be (or have been) a mother to you although they did not physically bring you into the world?

3. Anna was the first person in the New Testament to have been given the title "prophet." What made her actions so prophetic?

4. During our holy waiting, we also must prepare. Write down ways that you will prepare your mind, body, and spirit for the next place God is leading you.

Chapter 5: Mary's Hair Shared Her Testimony: John 12:1–8

1. What is your relationship to your hair?

2. Mary practiced extravagant love toward Jesus publicly. How do you show extravagant love for Jesus?

3. What was the significance of washing Jesus's feet with costly perfume? How would you feel about using something as intimate as the hair on your head to groom someone else's feet? If you are studying this book in a group, wash one another's feet as an act of extravagant love and hospitality.

Chapter 6: A Virgin's Life: Luke 1:26–38

1. How can you possess the liberated spirit of the Virgin Mary according to Renita Weems's definition of the word *virgin*?

2. Think about your faith walk. Consider the ways that as a twenty-first-century believer you can interpret your faith in a world where organized religion is less prominent. Write down your ideas.

3. How will you empower adolescent girls to know that their thoughts matter and to believe that they

can, even at a young age, surrender their lives to God and make an impact in the world?

4. We are now at the end of our study. Reconsider your goals when you began. God is saying to you that with God nothing will be impossible. Do you believe that? What will you accomplish in your life since there is no impossibility with God?

ABOUT THE AUTHOR

A minister, blogger, podcaster, and spiritual entrepreneur, Jaimie is a graduate of Wellesley College. She earned her Master of Divinity and Master of Sacred Theology degrees from Yale Divinity School. She was ordained to Christian Ministry in 2015, and her ordination is recognized by the American Baptist Churches, USA. Follow her work on her blog, I Am Free Agent.

Printed in the United States
By Bookmasters